THE
BOOK OF
IT

BEV AISBETT

HarperCollins*Publishers*

HarperCollins*Publishers*

First published in Australia in 2001
as *The Little Book of IT*
This format published in 2008
by HarperCollins*Publishers* Australia Pty Limited
ABN 36 009 913 517
www.harpercollins.com.au

HarperCollins*Publishers*
Level 13, 201 Elizabeth Street, Sydney NSW 2000, Australia
31 View Road, Glenfield, Auckland 10, New Zealand
77–85 Fulham Palace Road, London, W6 8JB, United Kingdom
2 Bloor Street East, 20th floor, Toronto, Ontario M4W 1A8, Canada
10 East 53rd Street, New York NY 10022, USA

National Library of Australia Cataloguing-in-Publication data:

Aisbett, Bev.
    The book of it: ten steps to conquer anxiety.
    2nd ed.
    ISBN 978 0 7322 8700 9 (pbk.).
    1. Anxiety. 2. Anxiety – Treatment. 3. Stress management. I. Title.
152.46

Illustrations by Bev Aisbett
Internal design adapted by Kirby Jones, and cover design adapted by
Matt Stanton from the original design by Raylee Sloan, kinart
Printed and bound in Australia by Griffin Press
50gsm Bulky used by HarperCollins*Publishers* is a natural, recyclable product
made from wood grown in sustainable forests. The manufacturing processes conform
to the environmental regulations in the country of origin, New Zealand.

9 8 7   12 13 14

PREFACE

Following the success of her books on anxiety, *LIVING WITH IT, LIVING IT UP* and *LETTING IT GO*, and *TAMING THE BLACK DOG* for depression, Bev Aisbett devised a workshop to further assist those with these conditions.

Since 1998, the WORKING WITH IT recovery program has assisted hundreds of people towards recovery from crippling anxiety.

This book outlines the ten basic steps which comprise the foundation for the workshops, and provides the basic tools with which you may build your own recovery.

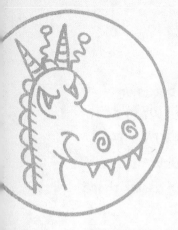

To all my students,
who have also been
my teachers

For further information on
anxiety, contact:

ANXIETY DISORDERS ASSOCIATION
OF VICTORIA (ADAVIC) 03 9853 8089 or
visit ADAVIC's website:
www.adavic.org

or visit BEV'S WEBSITE at
www.bevaisbett.com

CONTENTS

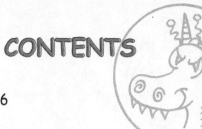

This is IT   6

THE TEN STEPS

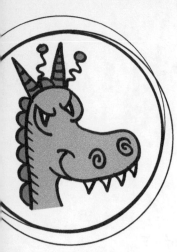

This is IT

In case you're not on
a first-name basis...

...this is "IT"!

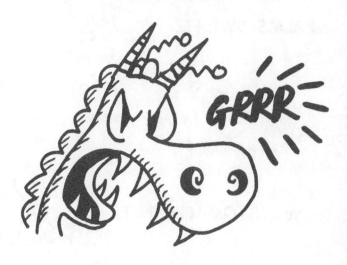

GRRR

He's responsible for bringing
you **PANIC ATTACKS**
and **ANXIETY**.

IT can be a bit of a handful...

IT can make your
PALMS SWEAT...

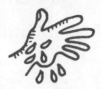

...your
HEART
race...

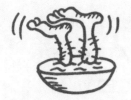

...your **STOMACH KNOT...**

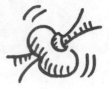

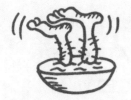

...and turn your
LEGS
to **JELLY!**

You probably think that you stumbled across your IT by *accident...*

...out of a **CLEAR BLUE SKY...**

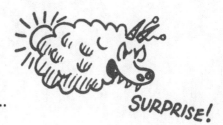

SURPRISE!

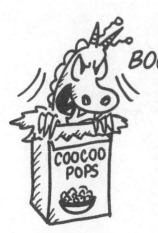

BOO!

...or in the **SUPERMARKET...**

...or at that
IMPORTANT
MEETING...

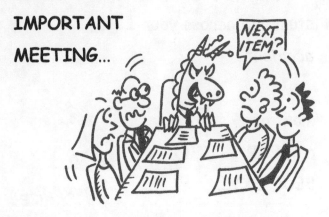

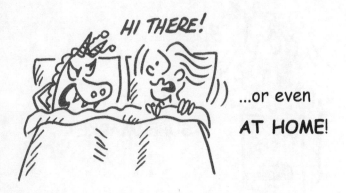

...or even
AT HOME!

The Book of IT

...and, because IT seemed to pop up
at *random*, you *never know* when he's
going to pop up again!

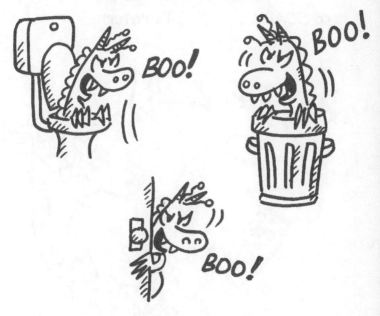

Naturally, that makes you
feel very **ANXIOUS**!

Now you're caught in a **LOOP**.

IT feels   ...you DREAD
so SCARY...   ITs return.

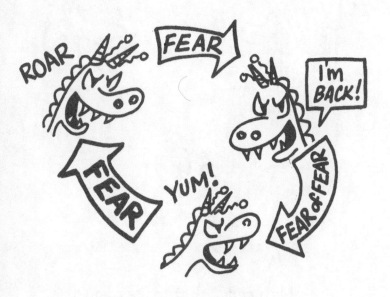

IT *GROWS!*   IT feeds
                   on FEAR.

So you feel <u>STUCK</u>.

You think...

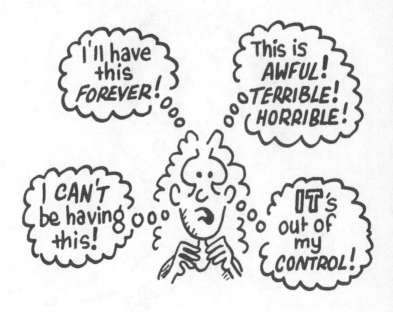

Talk about **SCARING** yourself!

But most of all, you ask...

WHY ME?

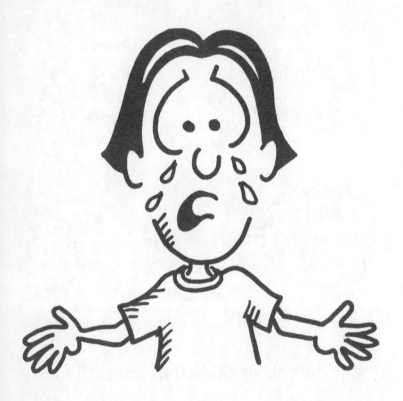

Well, let's answer that question.

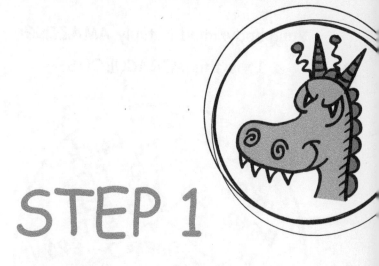

STEP 1

Understanding how you got your IT

Your body/mind is truly **AMAZING**!

It is this MIRACULOUS,

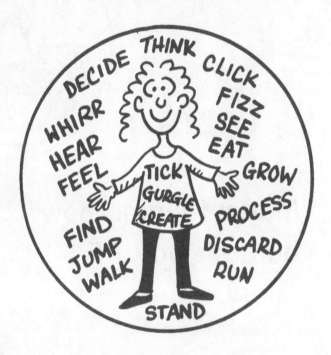

MARVELLOUS, totally

SELF-CORRECTING system.

Its aim is to keep you
BALANCED — no matter
WHAT you do to it!

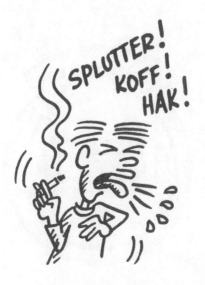

For instance,
if you SMOKE, you'll get a COUGH
which CLEANS OUT the **TOXINS**!

If you EAT the wrong
thing, it will CLEAR your
system of POISONS!

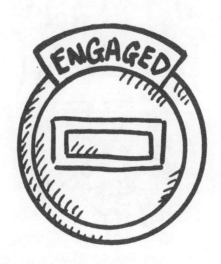

Your body/mind WANTS
TO KEEP YOU **HEALTHY**!

The symptoms that you have when your body is trying to reinstate balance might not be PLEASANT, but they are not intended to **HURT** you!

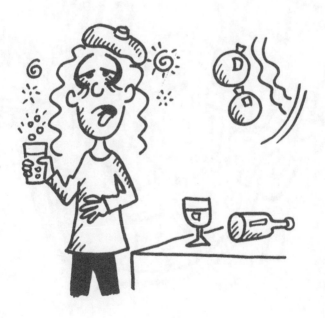

It's the same with your ANXIETY.
It is not a PUNISHMENT — IT
is a **WAKE-UP CALL!**

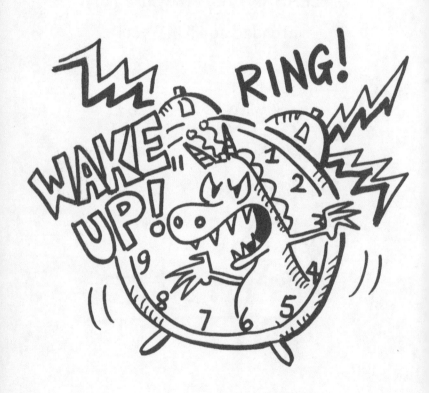

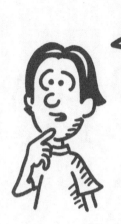

Well, I guess I <u>have</u> always been *HIGHLY STRUNG!*

Rather than anxiety being the BEGINNING of a problem, it is the END RESULT of years of accumulated PHYSICAL, MENTAL, EMOTIONAL and SPIRITUAL **STRESS**!

Basically, you're out of
BALANCE!

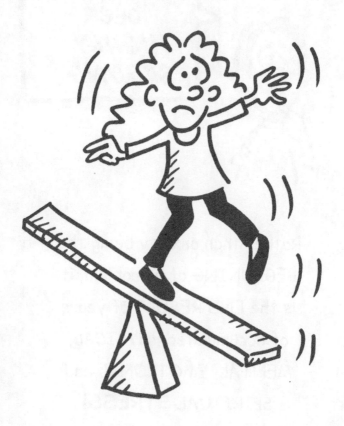

The Book of IT

TRY THESE QUESTIONS:

- Did you have a troubled childhood?
- Are there people you can never forgive?
- Do you put yourself down for mistakes?
- Do you often worry, worry, worry?
- Do you tend to expect the worst?
- Do things have to be perfect before you can enjoy them?
- Do you have a belief that life is hard?
- Are you concerned about what others think of you?

- Do you compare yourself to others?
- Do you have trouble expressing your feelings — especially anger?
- Do you give more than you get?
- Do you look after yourself as much as you do others?
- Are you critical of yourself and others?

If you answered "YES" to even HALF of these questions, would you say that your life and emotions are in BALANCE?

Look at it this way:
PHYSICAL fitness relies on keeping
things running smoothly, just like a
car.

A HEALTHY CAR

- SUITS YOUR
  NEEDS

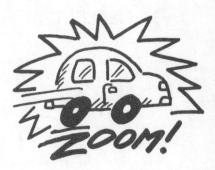

- GETS GOOD
  FUEL

- IS IN TUNE

- IS DRIVEN ONLY TO ITS LIMITS

- IS CARED FOR

AN UNHEALTHY CAR

- IS WRONG FOR YOUR NEEDS

- GETS ANY OLD FUEL

- IS OUT OF TUNE

- IS PUSHED TOO FAR

- IS NEGLECTED

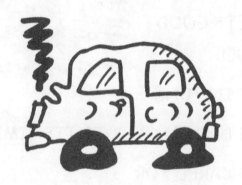

You are more than just a
PHYSICAL BEING, however.

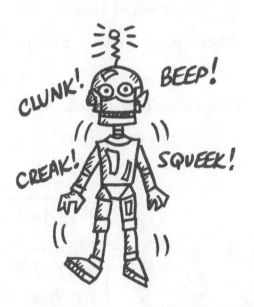

You also need EMOTIONAL,
MENTAL and SPIRITUAL
FITNESS to run your life
smoothly.

How much time have you spent
on TAKING CARE OF
or HEALING
these parts of your being?

How **HEALTHY** is your mind,
heart and spirit?

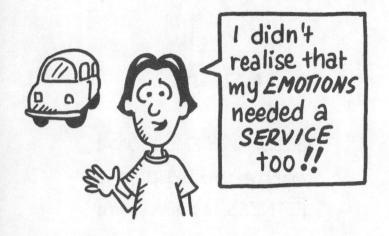

Given all this STUFF you've
been carting around, is it any
SURPRISE that you feel
ANXIOUS?

So, instead of asking...

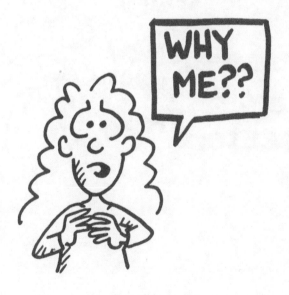

It might be more
REALISTIC to ask...

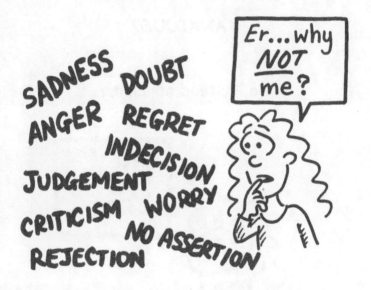

The Book of IT

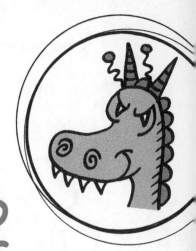

STEP 2

Accepting the
experience of IT

You can have a PROBLEM...

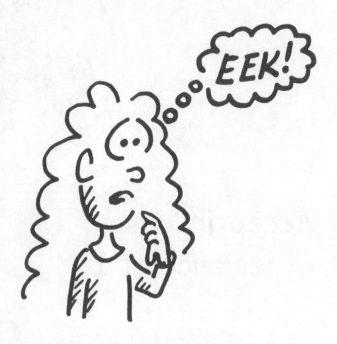

The Book of IT

...or you can have a **TERRIBLE HORRIBLE AWFUL TERRIFYING HIDEOUS** problem!

Just for NOW,
you are going through
an EXPERIENCE called **ANXIETY**.

There are **REASONS**
why you have arrived at this
experience of ANXIETY.

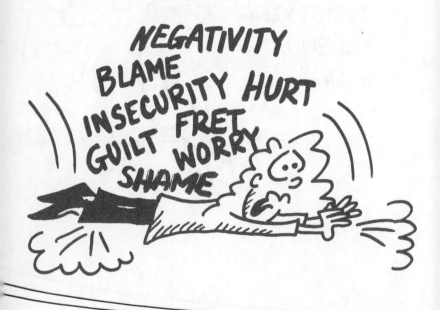

The Book of IT

Given your stressful approach to life, it's no great MYSTERY that this stress has tipped over into **ANXIETY!**

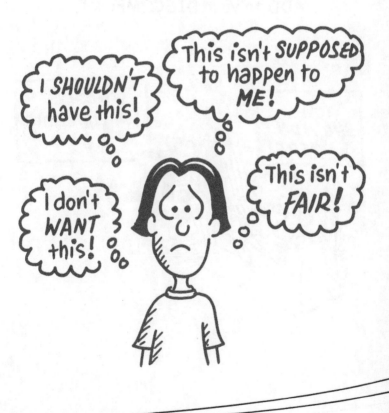

The more you **RESIST** being where you ARE, having what you're HAVING, feeling what you're FEELING, the more **PAIN** you will **ADD** to your DISCOMFORT.

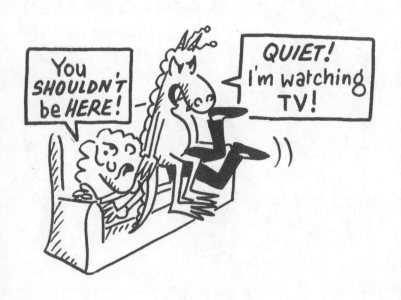

AND the more you add
AWFULISING to your
discomfort, the more
PAIN you will feel.

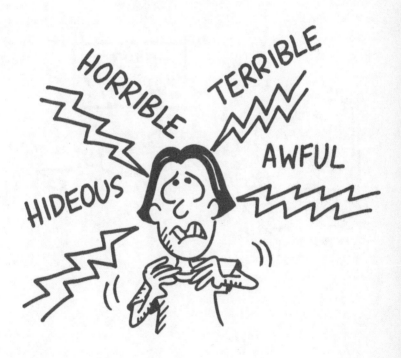

If you were PHYSICALLY rundown
and you came down with the 'flu,
you would ACCEPT that you have
the 'flu for a **REASON**.

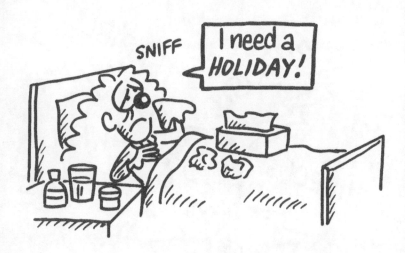

The Book of IT

And when you have the 'flu, you **ACCEPT** its symptoms as being part of the deal.

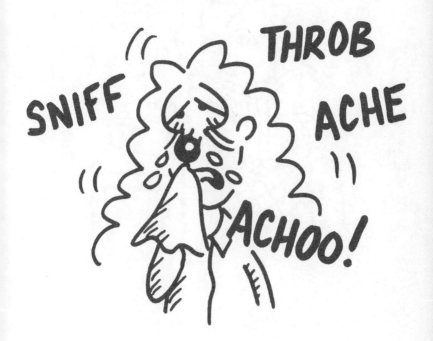

You WAIT IT OUT...

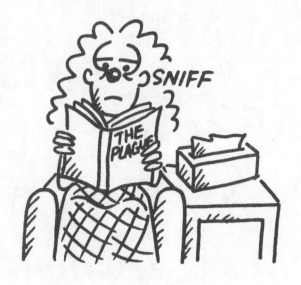

The Book of IT

...and then, if you're wise, you ATTEND to those factors that led you to be **VULNERABLE** in the first place!

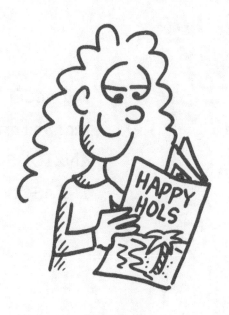

ACCEPTING the experience
of ANXIETY works in the
same way.

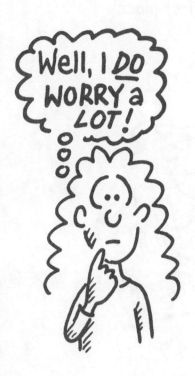

You ACCEPT
that you are
ANXIOUS for
a **REASON**.

And you ACCEPT that there
are certain SYMPTOMS that
go with ANXIETY.

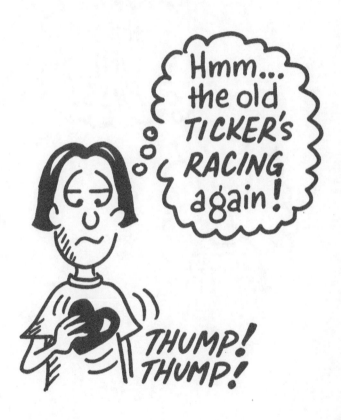

You WAIT IT OUT...

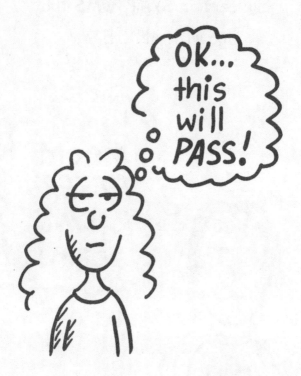

and then you ATTEND to
the things that CAUSED
you to be ANXIOUS.
(This book will help you do that.)

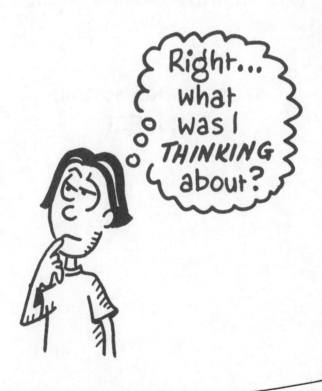

The **SYMPTOMS** you feel
are **PHYSICAL**. Any **THREAT**
you attach to them comes
from your **THINKING**.
(We'll do THINKING next chapter.)

THERE IS NO ACTUAL
DANGER!

INTERESTING FACT:

In some Eastern cultures,
certain meditation practices aim
to CREATE the very symptoms
you are doing your DARNEDEST
to get RID OF!

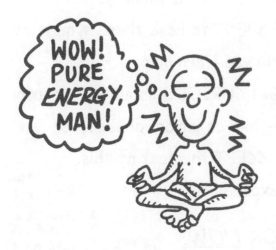

SAME SYMPTOMS BUT NO FEAR
OF THEM!

So, if you have a *dose* of anxiety...

- Let the SYMPTOMS just be SYMPTOMS
- Don't ADD to them with your THINKING
- Don't JUDGE them
- EXPECT to have these symptoms till you learn more
- Get CURIOUS about the symptoms — like an impartial observer
- ACCEPT the fact of this experience

FOR <u>NOW</u>.

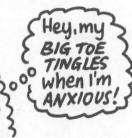

Hey, my BIG TOE TINGLES when I'm ANXIOUS!

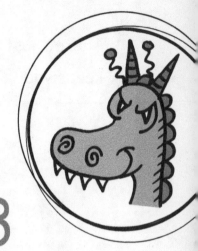

STEP 3

Handling your
IT thinking

There's just **ONE THING** that keeps you BOUND to your IT...

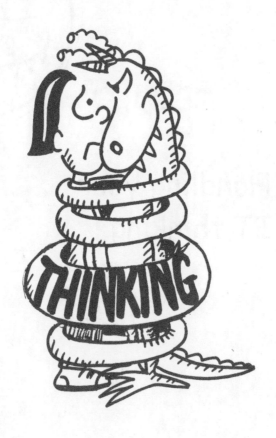

How can you expect **NOT** to feel
ANXIOUS...

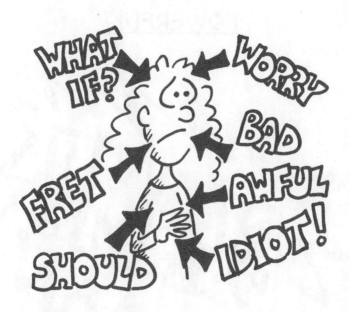

...if you keep **THINKING** in an
ANXIOUS way?

GET THIS...

YOUR THOUGHTS ARE
<u>POWERFUL!!</u>

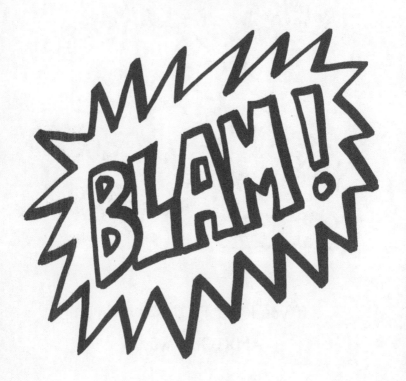

POWERFUL enough
to **CREATE** your IT!

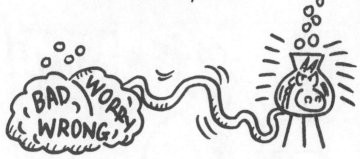

POWERFUL enough to
keep your IT **RUNNING**...

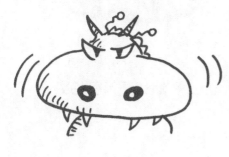

But also
POWERFUL
enough to
turn your IT
OFF again!

Your THOUGHTS are IT food!

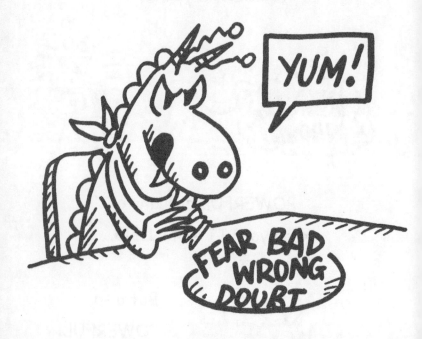

They feed your IT with ENERGY!

Feed IT enough and IT'll

EXPAND!

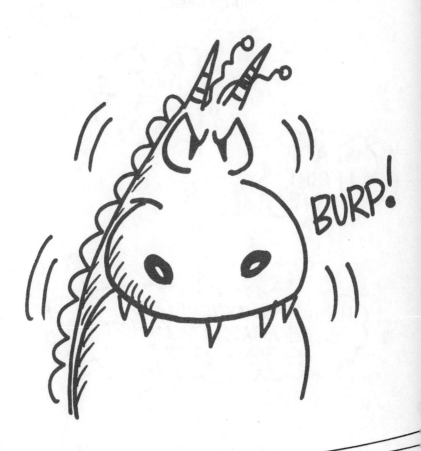

Beware of

IT JUNK FOODS

like these...

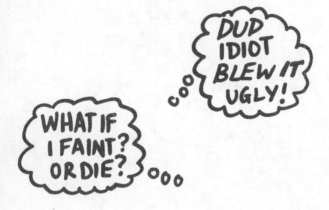

The Book of IT

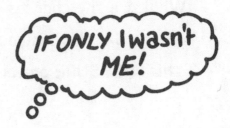

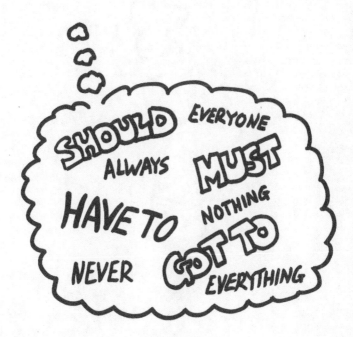

What are the chances of your feeling CALM when you put all this **PRESSURE** on yourself?

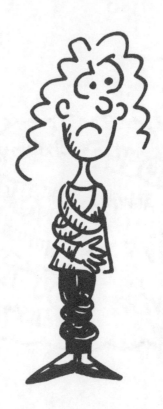

Turning around this THINKING
involves a **CHANGE OF MIND**.

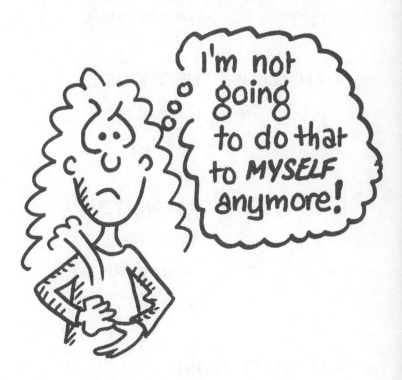

HERE'S WHAT TO DO:

1. MONITOR YOURSELF

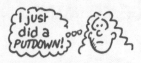 Be AWARE of
your self-talk.

2. CHALLENGE THE THOUGHT

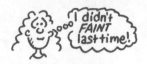 Is it based
on FACT?

3. CHOOSE AN ALTERNATIVE

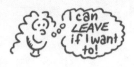 What thought
would SUPPORT
you?

4. LEAVE IT ALONE

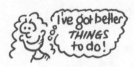 Do something else.
Cut the loop.

It takes **TIME** and **PRACTICE**
to turn around your IT thinking.

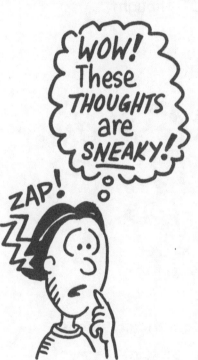

After all, most
of it has been
AUTOMATIC...

...But eventually, you'll feel a little *ZING!* when you stray into an IT thought...

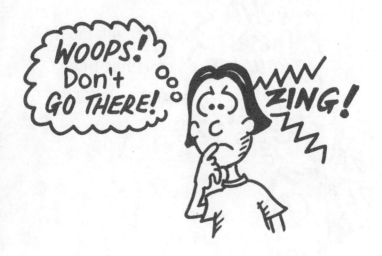

...and you'll automatically choose a HEALTHIER ALTERNATIVE. Best of all, as a result, your IT will gradually **SLIM DOWN**!

STEP 4

Watching for IT tricks

IT can be tricky, however.

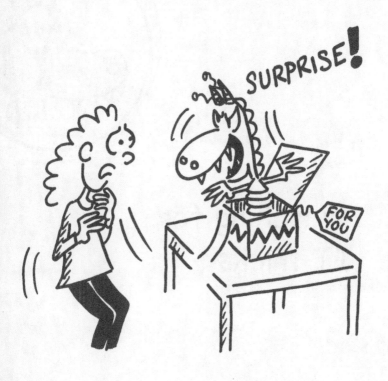

IT will try to convince you that
some things are *essential*...

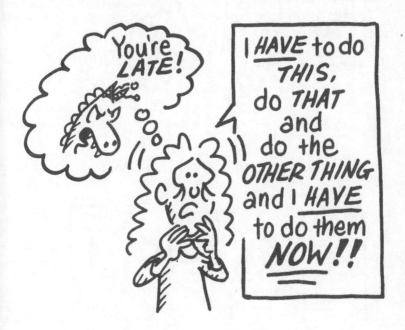

...such as lots of
DEADLINES...

...that you need to be **PERFECT**...

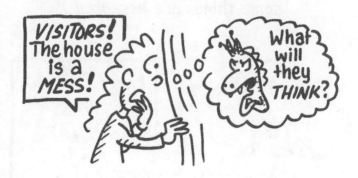

...and never make a **MISTAKE**!

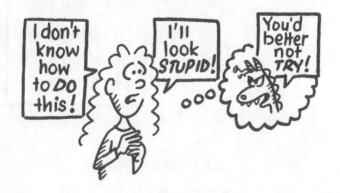

The Book of IT

IT will have you constantly
PREDICTING DISASTER...

What if I PANIC?

What if they see me PANIC?

What if I wear the WRONG THING?

What if I'm LATE?

CHEW CHEW

What if I FAINT?

What if I say the WRONG THING?

What if I make a FOOL of myself?

...and **RERUNNING THE PAST!**

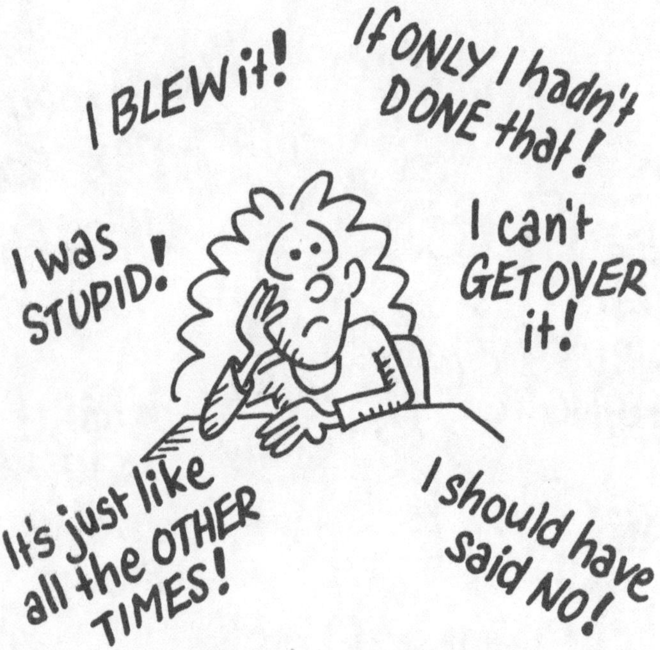

IT will tell you that you should be
APPROVED OF by **EVERYBODY**...

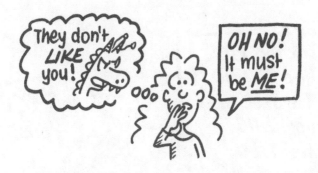

...that you should COMPARE
YOURSELF to **EVERYBODY**...

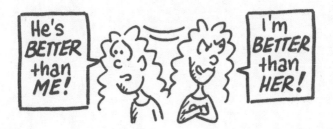

...and that you are never
GOOD ENOUGH!

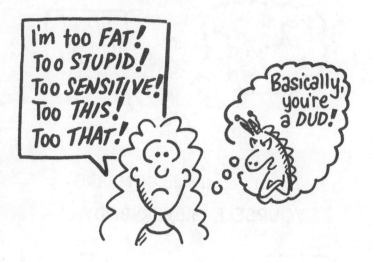

The Book of IT

IT will also con you into
BELIEVING that you are
RESPONSIBLE for **OTHERS'**
FEELINGS...

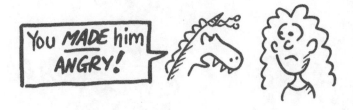

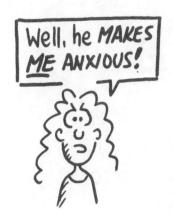

...or, worse...that
OTHERS have
control over how
YOU feel!

WRONG!!!

IT tricks are CREATED
by a set of **BELIEFS**...

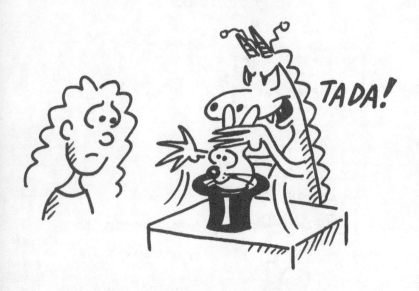

...and these BELIEFS
are based on **ILLUSIONS**!

And these *ILLUSIONS*
are based on **ONE THING**...

FEAR!

FEAR of being JUDGED

FEAR of being UNWORTHY

FEAR of DISAPPROVAL

FEAR of not BELONGING

FEAR of being VULNERABLE

FEAR of being REJECTED

FEAR of not being LOVED

and

FEAR OF FEAR!

What if you did not **FEAR**
these things?

And, above all, what if you
did not **FEAR** your IT?

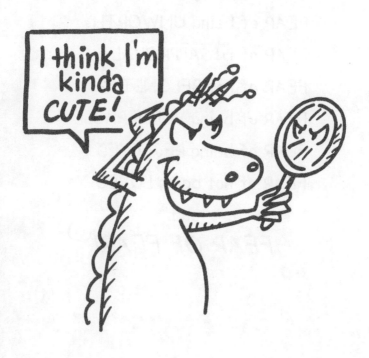

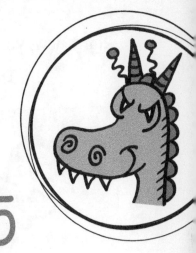

STEP 5

Working IT out

Right now, you don't like your IT.
In fact...

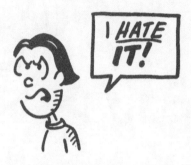

...you want IT GONE...*NOW!*

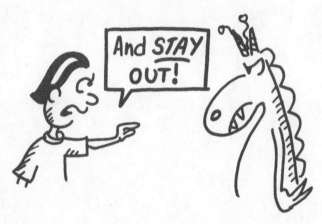

The Book of IT

But how can you get rid of IT
if you keep feeding IT **FEAR**?

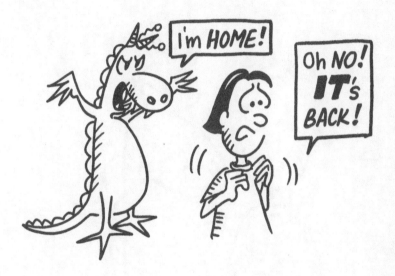

It might be time to rethink your
RELATIONSHIP with IT!

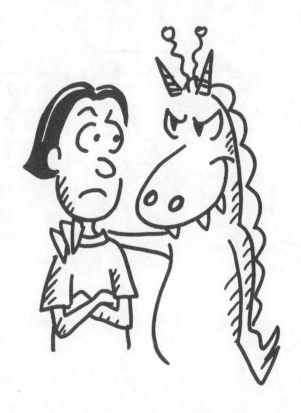

Perhaps IT serves a **PURPOSE**!

IT is telling you one
simple thing...

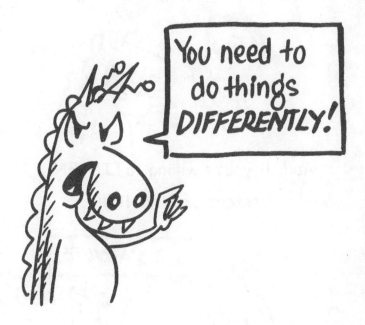

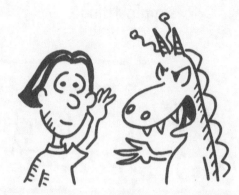

And...if you're willing to LISTEN...

...instead of RUNNING...

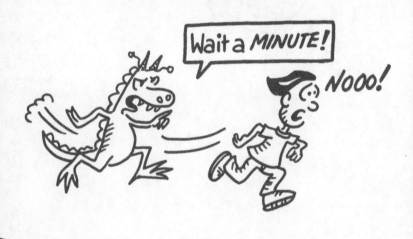

Wait a *MINUTE!*

NOOO!

...IT can act as a guide to
WHAT you need to do
DIFFERENTLY!

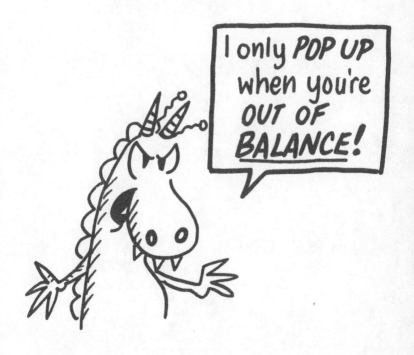

When you feel FEAR,

IT may be telling you to...

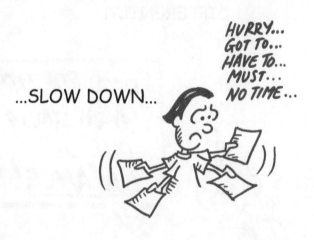

...SLOW DOWN...

HURRY...
GOT TO...
HAVE TO...
MUST...
NO TIME...

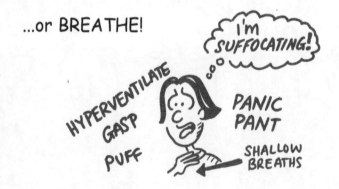

...or BREATHE!

I'm SUFFOCATING!

HYPERVENTILATE
GASP
PUFF

PANIC
PANT

SHALLOW
BREATHS

IT can warn you of...

...STINKY THINKING...

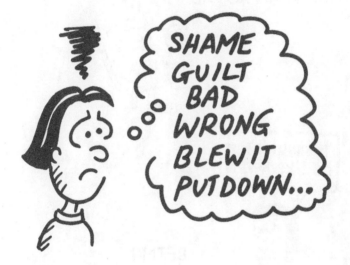

...or that you are...

...TRYING TO
WIN APPROVAL...

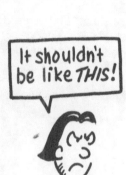

...BEING
INFLEXIBLE

And IT can alert you to...

NOT LIVING
IN THE
PRESENT...

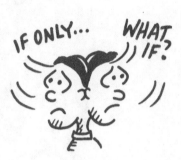

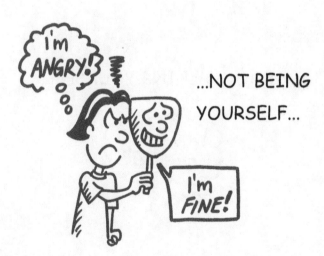

...NOT BEING
YOURSELF...

...OVERCONCERN FOR OTHERS'
OPINIONS...

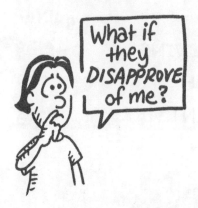

...and not VALUING YOURSELF.

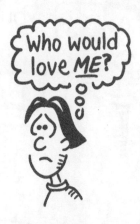

The Book of IT

IT is your guide to WHAT needs REBALANCING...

...and YOU work on the **HOW**!

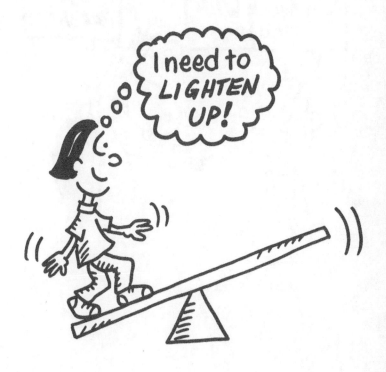

Now you're a **TEAM!**

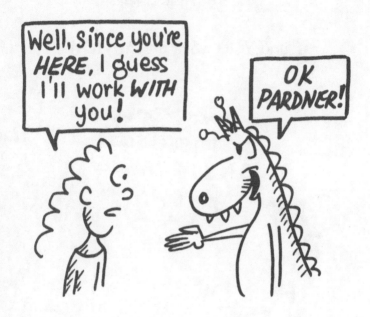

The Book of IT

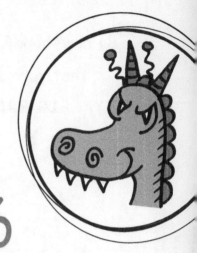

STEP 6

Finding what's behind IT

By now, hopefully, you are realising
that your **IT** is not really a
BIG BAD MONSTER...

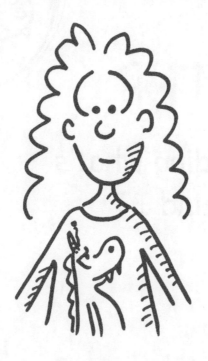

After all, your **IT** is part of **YOU**!

So, how did you and IT come to
decide that...

- Life is a STRUGGLE
- If I give LOVE, I get HURT
- I'm not GOOD ENOUGH
- I have to keep people HAPPY
- I can't show my FEELINGS
- It's scary to be POWERFUL
- I'm HELPLESS
- It's not OK to lose CONTROL?

Most of this goes WAY back...

...to the creation of little **IT**...

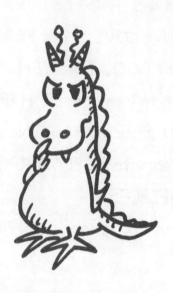

...through the

BELIEFS of **CHILDHOOD**!

CHILDHOOD is the
time when we learn...

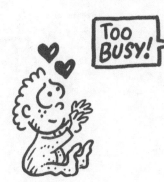

...how **LOVE**
works...

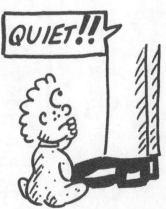

...how **POWERFUL**
PEOPLE behave...

...that **EXPRESSING** our
FEELINGS can be **WRONG**...

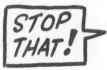

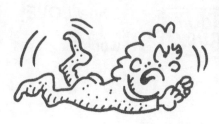

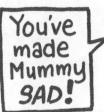

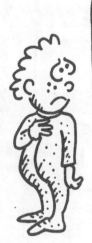

...and that our
BEHAVIOUR
affects **OTHERS**.

Children are,
by nature,
EGOCENTRIC...

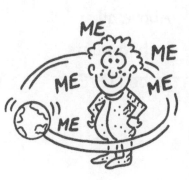

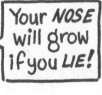
...they take
things
LITERALLY...

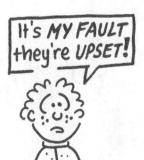
...and they
take things
PERSONALLY!

Above all,
a child wants
to be **LOVED**...

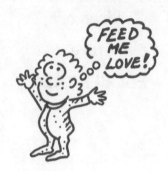

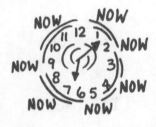

...24 hours a day...

...without
CONDITIONS!

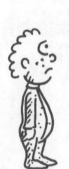

A child quickly learns how to gain
love or attention by being:

GOOD

QUIET

SICK

CLEVER

OBEDIENT

FUNNY

PLACID

HELPLESS and...WRONG!

Little by little, we learn that some parts of ourselves are **NOT OK**...

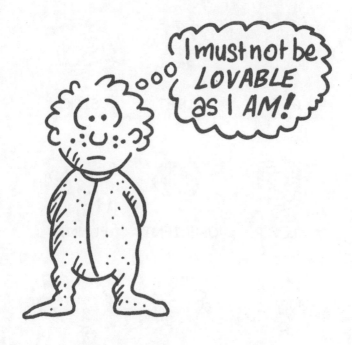

... because those parts aren't **LOVED** as much as other parts.

Even now, when you feel
ANXIOUS, you feel your
WORTH is on the line.

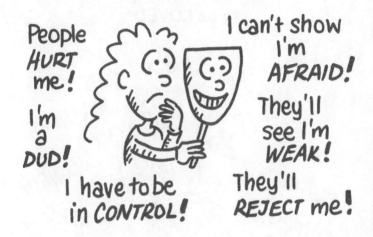

You fear those parts of you
that are not LOVABLE being
EXPOSED, just as you did
WAY BACK THEN.

Your **IT** is no more than
that little kid trying to
be **GOOD**, wanting
to be **LOVED**...

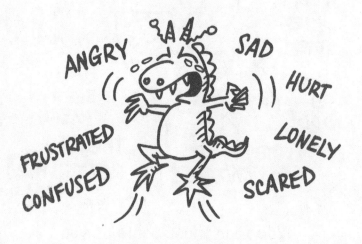

ANGRY SAD HURT

FRUSTRATED LONELY

CONFUSED SCARED

...but inside, all those
"unacceptable" feelings are
OUT OF CONTROL and that's
NOT LOVABLE!

STEP 7

Mending your
broken IT

So, how can you get your
ANGRY, NOISY, NASTY IT
back in line?

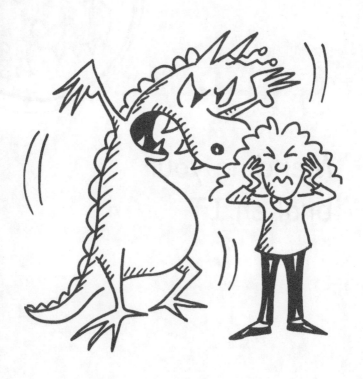

The Book of IT

If you think of your **IT** as an unruly **CHILD**, then you will need to employ some **TOUGH LOVE** to get back some peace and order.

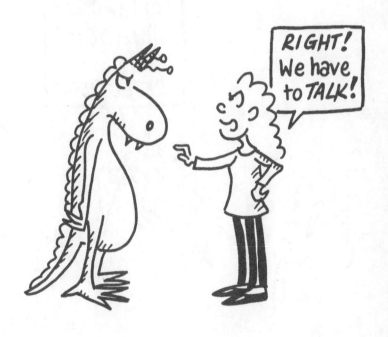

RIGHT! We have to TALK!

LISTEN

Your IT has been trying to tell you
what your REAL fear is.

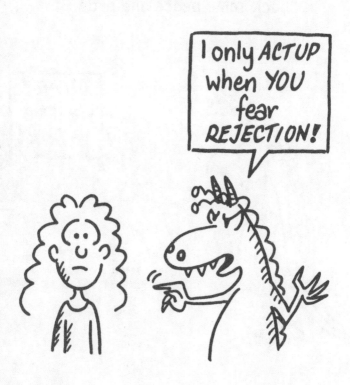

NEGOTIATE

Lay down some guidelines

for teamwork.

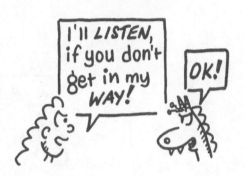

MONITOR

Your IT can
run amok if you
don't keep track of
old habits.

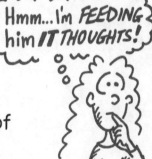

DISCIPLINE

Get back some ORDER and FOCUS
rather than INDULGING IT.

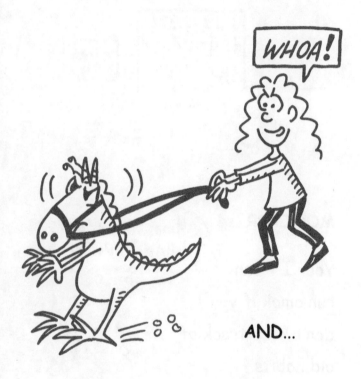

The Book of IT

...HEAL

Think of yourself as
the little child that
you were.

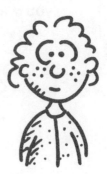

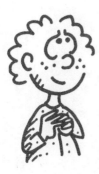

You just wanted
to be LOVED...

...you were SMALL...

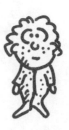

...you were **VULNERABLE**...

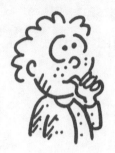

...you **TRUSTED**...

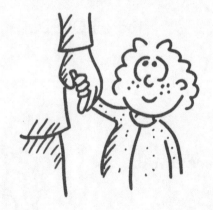

...you did the **BEST** you could...

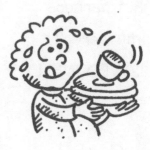

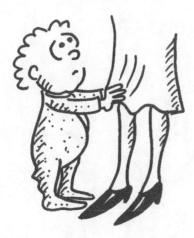

...and you tried to keep them happy.

But perhaps
you weren't
LOVED WELL...

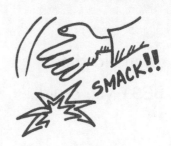

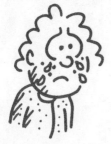

...you may have
been **HURT**...

...you may
have been
IGNORED...

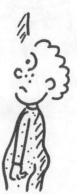

There may
have been
too many
RULES...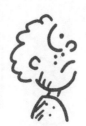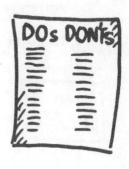

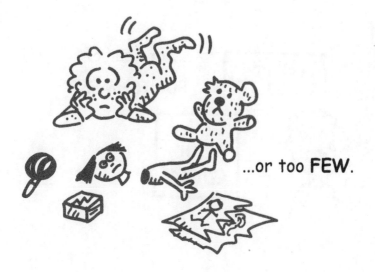

...or too **FEW**.

You may not have been able
to EXPRESS how you felt...

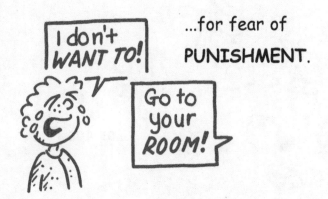

...for fear of
PUNISHMENT.

Or, because you were little,
you may have just
MISUNDERSTOOD.

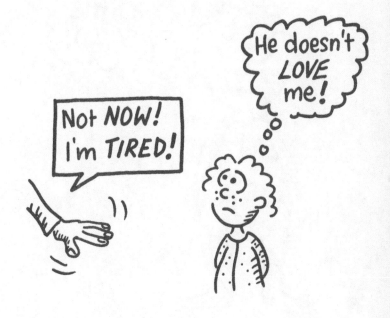

BUT...

...IT WASN'T YOUR **FAULT**.

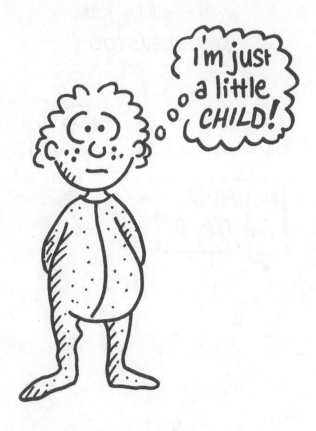

FORGIVE YOURSELF

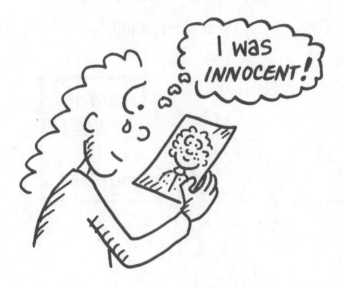

Give **YOURSELF** the love
you did not receive when
you were small.

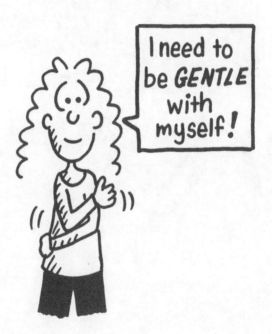

The Book of IT

AND...make **PEACE** with your **IT**...

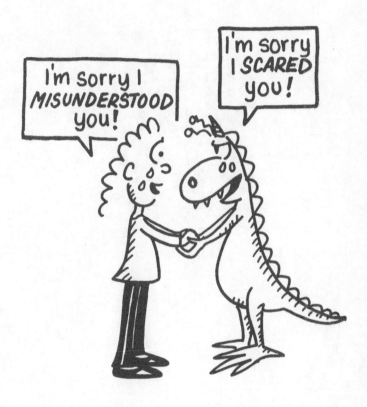

...he's just the little child in you.

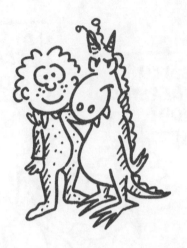

The Book of IT

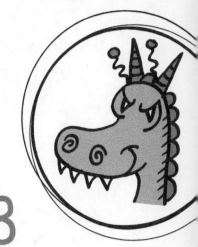

STEP 8

Healing your
relationship with IT
and others

Healing your relationship with
YOURSELF is **VITAL**...

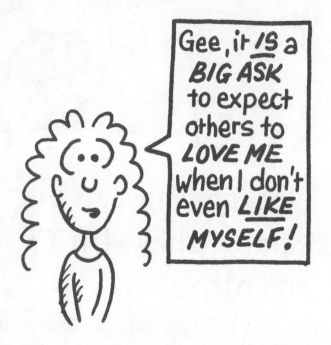

...and healing your
relationships with OTHERS
is the next important step.

So, who told you that you...

...were FLAWED
OR WRONG...

...needed to keep
EVERYBODY
HAPPY...

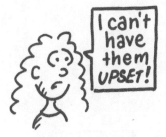

...or that you had
to be PERFECT?

SOMEONE must have...

...through
WORDS...

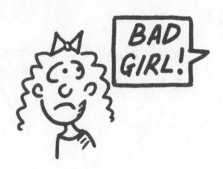

...or DEEDS.

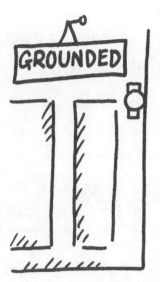

The Book of IT

In fact, you may have been
given this message over and
over in your life.

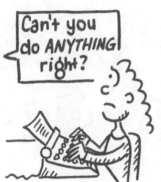
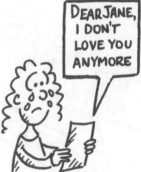

The thing is, no matter what
OPINION of you **OTHERS**
may have held...

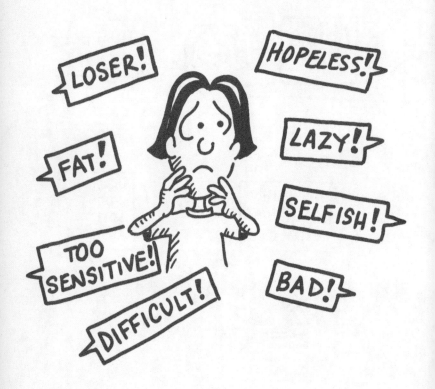

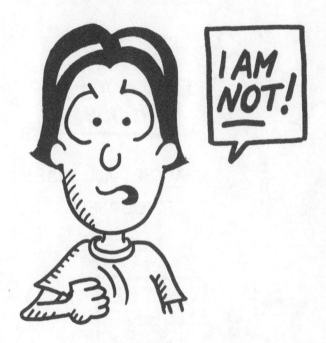

You can disagree if you...

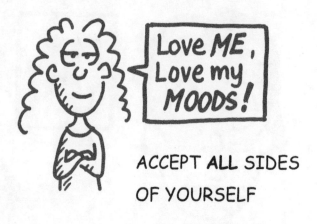

ACCEPT **ALL** SIDES
OF YOURSELF

STOP **APOLOGISING**
FOR BEING YOU

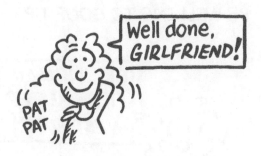

BE YOUR OWN **CHEER SQUAD,
DIRECTOR, COUNSELLOR
& FRIEND**

LOSE THE '**DISEASE TO PLEASE**'

BE WILLING TO **GOOF** UP

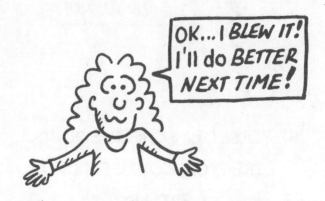

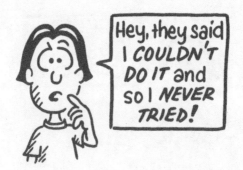

AND...STOP PROVING

THEM **RIGHT**!

But what if someone hurt you
TERRIBLY?

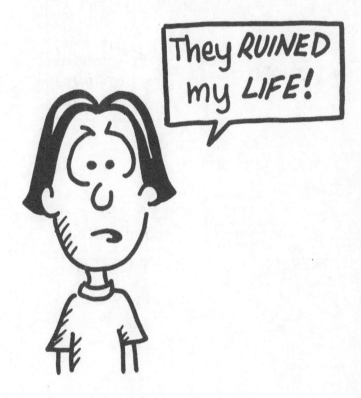

Again, you have **CHOICE**...

...to remain
WOUNDED...

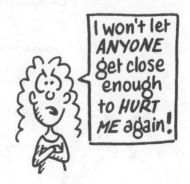

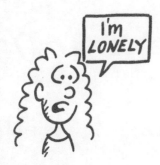

...and allow the
PAST to *KEEP*
hurting you...

...or to **DISCONNECT** from
the POWER that PAST events have
over you in the **PRESENT!**

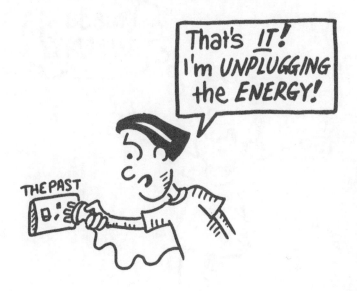

After all, the best REVENGE
is a **SUCCESSFUL LIFE!**

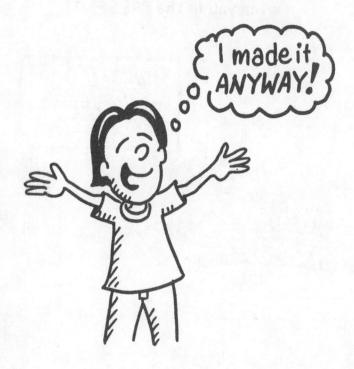

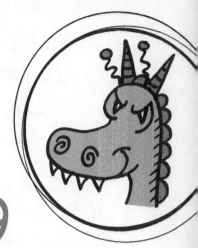

STEP 9

Transforming to an
IT-free outlook

So, what if there was less
to be UPSET, ANGRY or
WORRIED about?

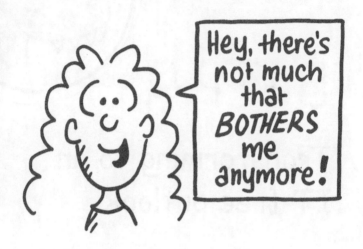

Wouldn't that mean
that you would feel
less **ANXIOUS**?

Most human misery comes from:

- NOT ACCEPTING THINGS AS THEY ARE

- NOT LIVING IN THE PRESENT

- RESISTING CHANGE

- REMAINING STUCK IN PAIN

- GIVING AWAY PERSONAL POWER

- TAKING LIFE PERSONALLY

Let's take a look at these:

- **NOT ACCEPTING THINGS AS THEY ARE**

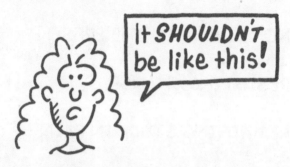

What if you looked for the OPPORTUNITY in ANY situation?

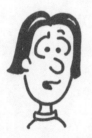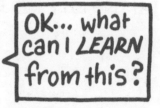

What if you had
FEWER EXPECTATIONS...

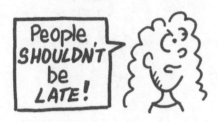

...and were more FLEXIBLE?

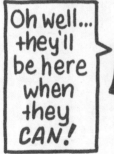 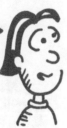

▪ NOT STAYING IN THE PRESENT

What if you
stopped
PREDICTING...

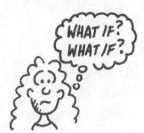

...and
REGRETTING...

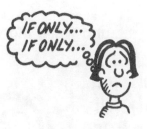

...and just dealt
with the HERE
and NOW?

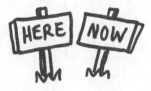

■ RESISTING CHANGE

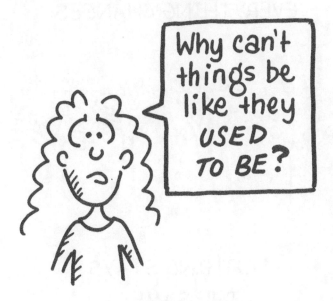

What if you planned for CHANGE
instead of PERMANENCE?

Think about it...

EVERYTHING CHANGES

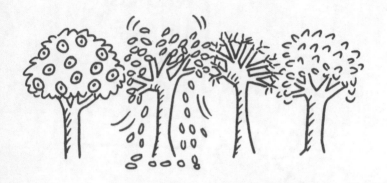

NOTHING STAYS
THE SAME...

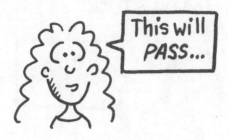

...and this can be a COMFORT
in the TOUGH times...

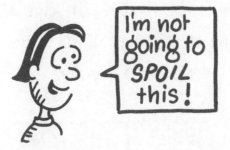

...and a reminder to CHERISH
the GOOD times.

▪ REMAINING STUCK

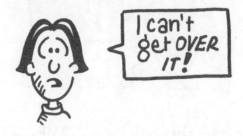

What if you saw PAIN as
a message to sort out some of
the things that NEED to be
SORTED anyway?

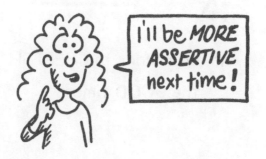

By using PAIN to make
some IMPROVEMENTS, you
TRANSFORM a NEGATIVE
into a POSITIVE.

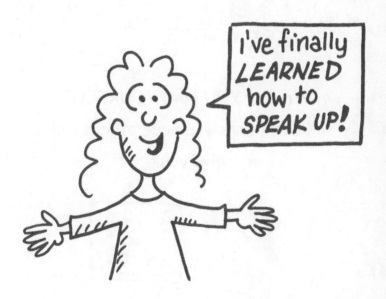

▪ GIVING AWAY POWER

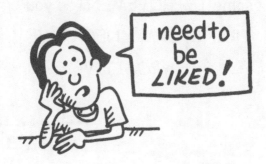

What if YOU gave YOURSELF
all the things you hope others will
give you?

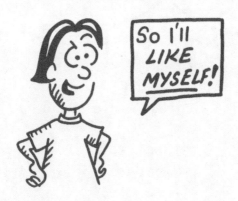

No-one can HURT you,
LET YOU DOWN or BETRAY
you if you don't give them the
POWER to do so!

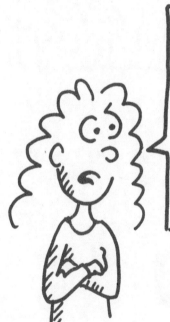

Hmm – he's
NEVER
been
TRUSTWORTHY!
It would be
UNWISE to
TRUST him!

What if you didn't give that
POWER away?

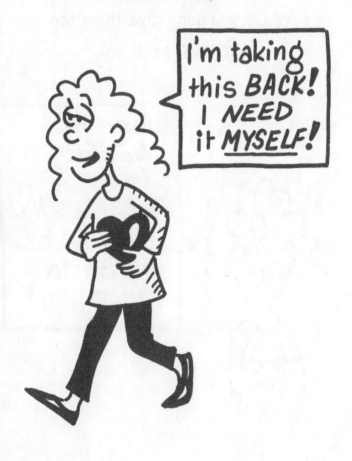

▪ TAKING LIFE PERSONALLY

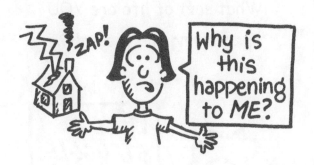

What if you didn't judge life as either FAIR or UNFAIR, but as a natural (and impartial) process?

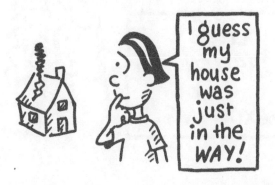

Life is what you PERCEIVE it to be.
What sort of life are YOU
perceiving for yourself?

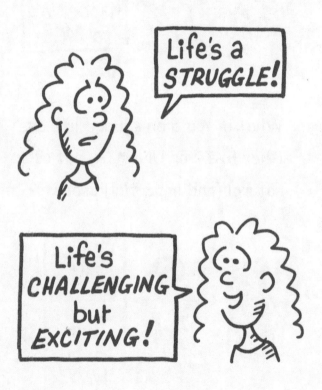

The Book of IT

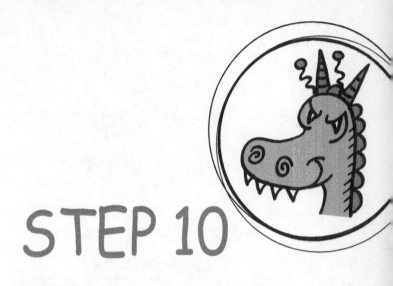

STEP 10

Moving beyond IT

Life can be a BUMPY RIDE
at times...

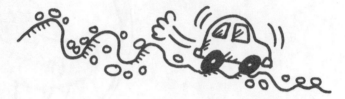

...but with a bit of care...

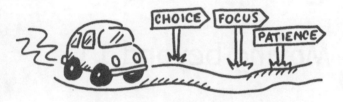

...the journey can smooth out.

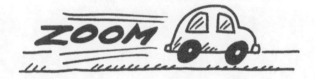

The thing is to have
CLEAR NAVIGATION
so you never STAY lost,
and a DESTINATION to
keep heading for!

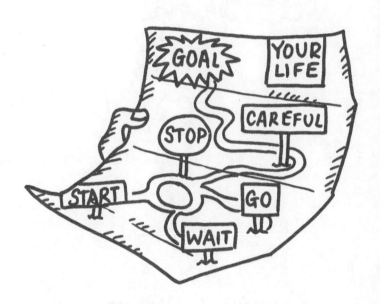

When you embark on this journey,
you get a TRAVELLING OUTFIT...

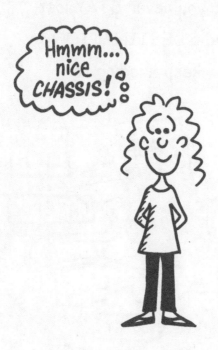

...your BODY, MIND and
PERSONALITY.

It may not *seem* to fit right at times, but it's a matter of making the necessary ADJUSTMENTS.

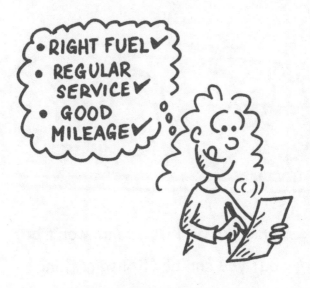

But it's yours for LIFE and it will fit much better if you TAKE CARE of it.

On this journey, you'll have some
PASSENGERS...

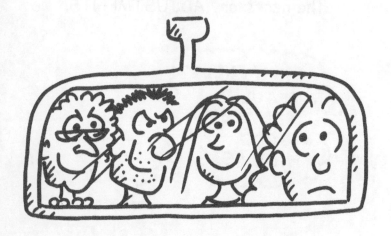

...some will be FUN, some won't be,
but you can LEARN something
about YOURSELF from
ALL of them.

Some may be HELPFUL...

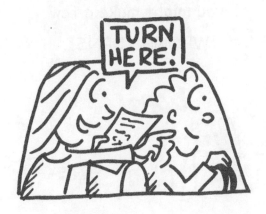

...but some may try to STEER you
in the **WRONG DIRECTION!**

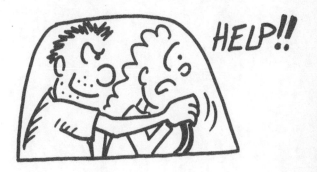

As you proceed on this journey,
you might make a few
WRONG TURNS...

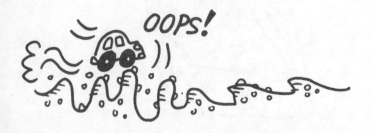

...especially while you're getting the
HANG OF IT...

...and if you don't take
a better route...

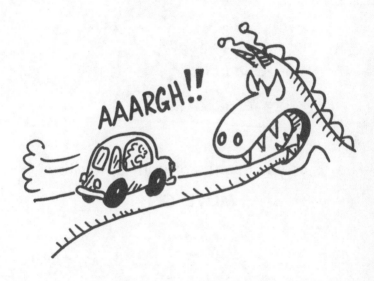

...you might end up running into a
MAJOR OBSTACLE!

At this point, you might **STALL**...

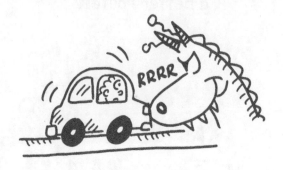

...or you might work out a way to

MOVE ON.

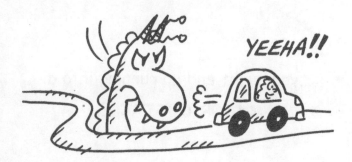

In either case, you will have learned
something valuable.

You will have learned
WHICH WAY
<u>NOT</u> TO GO AGAIN!

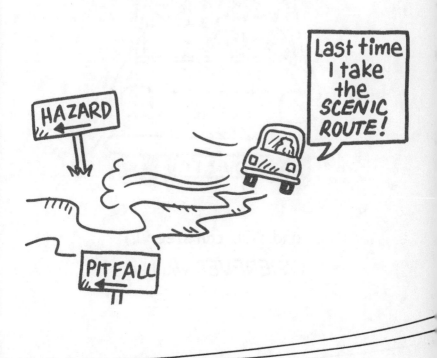

The bottom line is...

...it's *YOUR* journey...

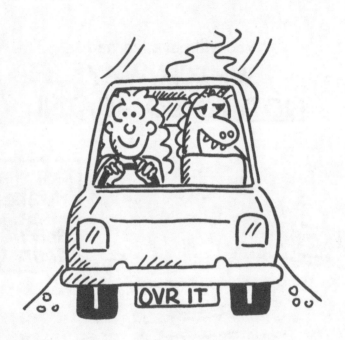

...and YOU can steer **IT**
WHEREVER you like!